LOSE YOUR BELLY FAT

SABAT BEATTO

Table of Contents

There are many dangerous and ineffective gimmicks about how to lose belly fat. While there's no "magic bullet" that will target abdominal fat in particular, this eBook has been specifically written to explain what causes an expanding waistline and how you can make that spare tire go away. You will be surprised by what you will learn.

It was on the second day of the New Year that I heard her saying "I can't do this; I just can't continue to live my life like this. I can't face another diet." Anastasia, my friend was making yet another series of desperate New Year's resolutions. "Every year, I starve myself for months, take different types of pills and supplements to lose maybe 4 inches off my waist, and in just few months it all comes back," she complained. "What's the point? I'm just not destined to have a flat tummy."

I understood how she felt. Obesity shortened my uncle's life, and for many years I struggled with a super puffy belly as well. I figured it was my genetic destiny to be bloated, too. But then I got sick and tired of being sick and tired, and I've made it my life's work to learn everything there is to know about obesity in general and belly fat in particular. In my many years as a health journalist I have come to discover many very important tips that will help to combat this menace of belly fat.

"What would you say if I told you that you can lose those belly fat once and for all just by following some simple steps?" I asked Anna. "What if you could lose much of that belly fat in just weeks?" You will be amazed by the many little things you have to do. Things you probably have ignored all this while because you never knew they actually work.

Overweight does not necessarily equal unhealthy. There are actually plenty of overweight people who are in excellent health. Conversely, many normal weight people have the metabolic problems associated with obesity. That's because the fat under the skin is actually not that big of a problem (at least not from a health standpoint… it's more of a cosmetic problem). It's the fat in the abdominal cavity, the belly fat that causes the biggest issues. If you have a lot of excess fat around your waistline, even if you're not very heavy, then you should take some steps to get rid of it.

Most women hate to even have an inch or so too much belly fat. How do you know, however, if the belly fat you carry is a health risk? Just measure it. Calculate your waist-to-hip ratio. Your waist-to-hip ratio

— or the circumference of your waist divided by the circumference of your hips — can be a good indicator of whether you need to lose belly fat. Here's how to get it:

- Wrap a soft tape measure around the thinnest part of your waist at the level of your navel. Note the measurement. Wrap the tape measure around the widest part of your hips, where you can feel a bony protrusion about 1/3 of the way from the top of the hipbone. Note the measurement.
- Divide your waist measurement by your hip measurement. Know what's healthy. Women should have a ratio of 0.8 or below; men should be at 0.9 or lower. Anything different from this is known as abdominal obesity

Abdominal obesity, also known as central obesity, is something that many people worldwide have problems with. Once you hit middle age, far too many people are plagued by those two dreaded words…belly fat. It can, however, also be a problem for children and teens. People just look at it as a weight problem, but it can also be linked to cardiovascular disease, Alzheimer's disease, and many other metabolic and vascular diseases.

Though no one likes belly fat, too often it is overlooked as just a symptom of age. It can, however, be a symptom of much, much more. It is not something you should just consider the price of getting older. It is something that should be taken seriously.

What is Belly Fat?

Belly fat is maligned for its way of tampering with any outfit that doesn't involve a muumuu, but really there's something way worse about the stuff: When white fat expands in your abdomen, nestling deep among your organs, it sets you up for some serious health trouble. We now know that this type of fat, called visceral fat, churns out stress hormones like cortisol and inflammatory substances called cytokines that affect the body's production of insulin. The result: It's worse than just being generally overweight; you're looking at increased risks of type 2 diabetes and cardiovascular disease.

Usually, belly fat is subcutaneous fat, which is underneath the skin. This is also known as organ fat because it is packed between your internal organs. This is also known as the "pot belly" or the "beer belly." It is associated with many health problems, even colorectal cancer.

In recent studies, scientists have come to realize that it isn't really how much a person weighs—it's their amount of body fat that truly indicates obesity. Throughout the 1980's and 90's imaging techniques were developed that helped improve the understanding of exactly how many health risks can be associated with the accumulation of body fat. These include tomography and magnetic resonance which help divide masses of tissue in the abdominal region.

For women, belly fat is more common after menopause. Sometimes people just think this goes hand-in-hand with getting older, and don't realize the danger it can cause. While women feel like it is just something that makes them go up a size in their jeans, it does carry health risks.

Like fat in any other area, it is determined by balancing the calories you take in with the energy you burn. In other words, if you eat too much and burn too little, you'll have excess fat. As you get older, your muscle mass reduces. Your fat, however, increases. When your muscle mass reduces, it also reduces the rate your body uses calories. This can make it even more difficult for people to maintain a weight that is healthy as they age.

Sometimes, you can have an increase of belly fat as you age without even gaining weight. In women, this can be due to a reduced level of estrogen. Research has shown that estrogen seems to influence where the fat is distributed in a woman's body. Regardless of a weight shown as normal on the BMI measurement charts, women with a large waistline have been known to carry the risk of premature death and often die earlier of cardiovascular disease.

.

People who are plagued with belly fat often exercise and participate in healthy activities, yet they still retain that unwanted fat. It seems like the fat is immune to exercise. So how do you get rid of it? What is the magic combination that says "poof" to that extra poundage? It depends on your sex, age, and the amount of pounds you want to lose, but there are many tips to help you reduce that unwanted belly fat.

Benefits of Losing Weight

Surprise: Everyone has some belly fat, even people who have flat abs. That's normal. But too much belly fat can affect your health in a way that other fat doesn't. Some of your fat is right under your skin. Other fat is deeper inside, around your heart, lungs, liver, and other organs. It's that deeper fat -- called "visceral" fat -- that may be the bigger problem, even for thin people.

Another surprise: Everybody needs some visceral fat. It provides cushioning around your organs. But if you have too much of it, you may be more likely to get high blood pressure, type 2 diabetes, heart disease, dementia, and certain cancers, including breast cancer and colon cancer. The fat doesn't just sit there. It's an active part of your body, making "lots of nasty substances," says Kristen Hairston, MD, assistant professor of endocrinology and metabolism at Wake Forest School of Medicine.

Being overweight isn't always easy, and as a result, it can have a negative effect on your self-esteem. It is, however, important for you to maintain the normal weight for more than cosmetic reasons. You need to maintain the proper weight for many health reasons. In a society like ours, where people put such an importance on the way we look, feeling unattractive can lead to serious depression. While is it that not all overweight people get depressed? Some are, in fact, quite happy the way they are, but many others can't handle the social stigma. It can lead to serious emotional and mental problems in addition to the other health problems.

It can be difficult to determine how much weight you need to lose to be healthy. You should realize, however, that you don't have to lose weight if you're not actually overweight.   More important than weight, is the amount of fat content you have in your body and where that fat has accumulated. Sometimes, you have weight gain because you've started working out and developed muscles. Muscles are heavier than fat, so don't be shocked if all that exercise has only reduced belly fat by inches but also increased weight. If this is the case, there's no problem at all and you don't have to worry about losing that weight.

While being too worried about our weight can be a problem too, knowing you're overweight and taking the steps to reduce that weight is important. There are many benefits to losing weight.
Here are a few of them:

- Reduces your risk of long-term health problems that could shorten your life. These include health problems such as diabetes and cardiovascular disease. Usually, this is the main reason most people try to lose weight.

- Feeling better, healthier, and having more energy. You'll be able to take the stairs, or walk from the far end of the parking lot without losing your breath.

- Less pain in your joints. Problems such as osteoarthritis in your knees and pain and swelling in your ankles can greatly be reduced. Being overweight puts a strain on them that you will feel greatly reduced when you lose weight.

- Many times when you lose weight, especially if you're diabetic or have high blood pressure, your doctor will be able to take you off your medication. Not only will you be healthier and not taking so much medication, you'll save a lot of money at the pharmacy counter.

- You'll feel better about yourself as you gradually join the people with smaller midsections. Your self-esteem will increase. You'll find yourself interacting with others in a whole new way.

- When you are eating out with co-workers you won't be overeating, because it has serious implications on the advancement of your career. Believe it or not, behavioral science specialists have studied this, and they found that eating healthy gives you the impression of a person that is outcome driven. This is something supervisors look for. When they see it in you, they take a closer look at you as an employee. Don't be surprised if you're looked at for a promotion you never thought you'd get.

- Save money—this is a given. If you eat less, naturally you won't be buying as much food when you eat out and when you eat at home. You'll save money all the way around. You could even put aside the extra money you normally spend on food. When your weight loss is complete, you could have enough money for a whole new wardrobe or a nice vacation to treat yourself. After all, you have worked hard, so you deserve a treat.

- Keep your sex drive and be more satisfied sexually—this is especially true for men. Studies has shown that show if a man is around 30 pounds overweight, he can have testosterone levels of a man that is at least 10 years older. This reduces their sex drive. There have also been studies that show that people who are obese are much less satisfied with their sexual experiences. Sex is an important part of your life, especially for those in a relationship. You want to get the most out of it. Stay fit and you will.

- You can have more friends—face it…overweight people can sometimes be outcasts. Sometimes, it's self-inflicted, but other times, people just stay away from the "fat" person. When you lose weight, you'll feel more like making friends. You'll be able to participate in more activities which will allow you to meet more people. You'll make friends from circles you didn't dream of before.

- Influence others—sometimes, especially in spouses, one losing weight can be a positive influence on others and cause them to lose weight as well. If your children are overweight as well, it could be a genetic issue. Influencing them to begin losing weight before it gets as "out of control" as it is for you can give them a head start on the genetic problem and like Barney says, "Nip it!"

As you have read earlier in this book, getting rid of your belly bulge is important for more than just vanity's sake. Excess abdominal fat—particularly visceral fat, the kind that surrounds your organs and puffs your stomach into a "beer gut"—is a predictor of heart disease, type 2 diabetes, insulin resistance, and some cancers. If diet and exercise haven't done much to reduce your pooch, then your hormones, your age, and other genetic factors may be the reason why. These are the possible reasons why your belly fat hasn't budged:

You have been doing the wrong workout

A daily run or Spin class is great for your heart, but cardio workouts alone won't do much for your waist. "You need to do a combination of weights and cardiovascular training," says Sangeeta Kashyap, MD, an endocrinologist at Cleveland Clinic. Strength training increases muscle mass, which sets your body up to burn more fat. "Muscle burns more calories than fat, and therefore you naturally burn more calories throughout the day by having more muscle," says Kate Patton, a registered dietitian at Cleveland Clinic.

You have been eating too many processed foods

"Refined grains like white bread, crackers, and chips, as well as refined sugars in sweetened drinks and desserts increase inflammation in our bodies," says Patton. "Belly fat is associated with inflammation, so eating too many processed foods will hinder your ability to lose belly fat." Natural foods like fruits, vegetables, and whole grains are full of antioxidants, which have anti-inflammatory properties and may therefore actually prevent belly fat, Patton says.

You have been eating the wrong fats

The body doesn't react to all fats in the same way. Research correlates high intake of saturated fat (the kind in meat and dairy) to increased visceral fat, says Patton. On the other hand, monounsaturated fats (the kind in olive oil and avocados) and specific types of polyunsaturated fats (mainly omega-3s, found in walnuts, sunflower seeds, and fatty fish like salmon) have anti-inflammatory effects in the body, and if eaten in proper portions may do your body good. But Patton warns that eating too much fat of any kind increases your calorie intake and could lead to weight gain, so enjoy healthy fats in moderation.

Your workout hasn't been challenging enough

To banish stubborn belly fat, you have to ramp up your workouts. In a study published in the journal Medicine and Science in Sports and Exercise, people who completed a high-intensity workout regimen lost more belly fat than those who followed a low-intensity plan. (In fact, the low-intensity exercises experienced no significant changes at all.) "You need to exercise at full intensity because the end goal is to burn more calories, and high intensity exercise does just that," says Natalie Jill, a San Diego, California.-based certified personal trainer. High intensity workouts mean you're going all out for as long as you can. If this sounds intimidating, think of it this way: you'll burn more calories in less time.

You have been doing the wrong exercises

Doing crunches until the cows come home? Stop it! When you're down to your final inches of belly fat, the dreaded crunch won't be the exercise that finally reveals your six-pack. "You can't spot reduce," Jill says. Instead, she suggests doing functional exercises that use the muscles in your core—abdominals, back, pelvic, obliques—as well as other body parts. "These exercises use more muscles, so there is a higher rate of calorie burn while you are doing them," she says. Planks are her favorite functional exercise—they activate not just your core muscles but also your arm, leg, and butt muscle.

Also try these exercises to focus on your core muscles:

Do the bridge: Get into the position for doing a push up/press up. Rest on your elbows and always keep your eyes to the floor. Pull your stomach muscles in tight, imagining them going to your backbone. As you do this, your bottom should be down and your back straight. Hold this position for as long as it feels comfortable. During the holding period, don't arch your back but keep it as straight as possible. If it feels too hard at first, allow your knees to form a resting platform. Aim to hold the position for 30 seconds and repeat this exercise 3-5 times.

Do squats: Stand with your feet 8–9 inches (20.3–22.9 cm) apart, extend your arms in front of you and squat your hips backward. Do four sets of 15-20 squats, working several minutes at a time.
Stretch the sides of your waist. Stand up straight, with your feet hip-width apart. Put your right hand on your right hip, and lift your left arm straight up, so that your palm faces to the right. Keeping your legs centered, lean to the right and "reach" over with your left arm, stretching your left side. Do 3-5 times on each side.

You have been stressed

Whatever your source of stress, be it tight deadlines, bills, your spouse, your kids—having too much of it may make it harder for you to drop unwanted pounds, especially from your middle. And it's not just because you tend to reach for high-fat, high-calorie fare when you're stressed, though that's part of it. It's also due to the stress hormone cortisol, which may increase the amount of fat your body clings to and enlarge your fat cells. Higher levels of cortisol have been linked to more visceral fat.

You may have been sick

If your testosterone levels are high—something that can occur with polycystic ovary syndrome (PCOS)—losing weight may be problematic. "If you're an apple shape and overweight, it's a good idea to see your doctor," Dr. Kashyap says, since there may also be a chance that you are prediabetic or diabetic.

If you tend to pack the pounds around your middle rather than your hips and thighs, then you're apple shaped. This genetic predisposition means ridding yourself of belly fat will be harder, Dr. Kashyap says, but not impossible.

You have been unmotivated

Are you committed to the work needed to lose belly fat? "Reducing belly fat takes a combination approach of a low-calorie diet that is high in fiber and low in carbohydrates and sugar along with cardiovascular and weight training," Dr. Kashyap says. "If you are willing to do the work, you can move past genetics and lose it."

You have been skimping on sleep

If you're among the 30% of Americans who sleep less than six hours a night, here's one simple way to whittle your waistline: catch more Zs. A 16-year study of almost 70,000 women found that those who slept five hours or less a night were 30% more likely to gain 30 or more pounds than those who slept 7 hours. The National Institutes of Health suggest adults sleep seven to eight hours a night.

You're getting older

As you get older, your body changes how it gains and loses weight. Both men and women experience a declining metabolic rate, or the number of calories the body needs to function normally. On top of that, women have to deal with menopause. "If women gain weight after menopause, it's more likely to be in their bellies," says Michael Jensen, MD, professor of medicine in the Mayo Clinic's endocrinology division. In menopause, production of the hormones estrogen and progesterone slows down. Meanwhile, testosterone levels also start to drop, but at a slower rate. This shift in hormones causes women to hold onto weight in their bellies. The good news: you can fight this process.

Fortunately, belly fat can be eliminated or reduced by the same means that other fat can. It just takes the right combination of diet and exercise. There are, however, other factors that can hinder weight loss and cause you to retain belly fat. Ready to lose your gut and get rid of love handles once and for all? We offer up 57 easy, doable (and yes, even fun) ways to shed fat—without cutting out fries or running stairs from now until doomsday.

The average man's body houses 43.2 pounds of fat. And at any one moment, that number is either increasing or decreasing—it's never stagnant. Spend more of each day burning fat than you do storing it, and over time, you'll bury your belly forever. Sound simple? It is. You see, there's no single secret formula for losing fat. In fact, find 50 successful losers and they'll give you 50 different ways to win the battle of the bulge. But we did them five better. On the following pages, you'll find 55 tips designed to help you lose your love handles, bust your gut, and define your abs. Simply incorporate three or four into your life every day, and you'll finish off your fat easier and faster than you ever imagined possible.

As you go on with these tips, do the following to help with your motivation:

- Continue taking your measurements as you progress: While incorporating the strategies below, keep measuring so you can see your progress.
- Weigh yourself at the same time each day: Because body weight fluctuates depending on the time of day, when you last ate or when you last had a bowel movement, standardize the process by weighing yourself at the same time each day. Many people choose to do this the first thing in the morning, before breakfast.

Below are 55 tips that can help you reduce belly fat and have that abs you've always dreamed of:

1.   Avoid Stress

Our bodies produce hormones in response to stress, research has found. One of these is cortisol. It will push your body to look for high-calorie food because it thinks it used a lot of its energy handling something that was stressful. It's kind of like tricking your body into thinking it's had a big workout, when in fact, it's done nothing but become anxious and upset. Years ago, eating that type of high-calorie food was fine when you were stressed, because you used more energy every day working in the fields or on farms. Our ancestors remained thin during stressful times because of their hard work.

Now, many of us live more sedentary lives. We simply can't burn that type of fat intake any longer. When you're under a large amount of chronic stress, it signals your body to keep on making cortisol. It becomes a vicious cycle. Gaining weight makes you even more stressed, so you produce more cortisol and eat more fattening foods.

You can reduce stress by doing several things. You can get more sleep. The average adult should get at least seven hours of sleep a night. You should keep things that are stressful away from the area you use for sleeping. Don't do work in bed if you can help it. That area should be for relaxation and rest instead of work. Simply work at leaving your worries outside the bedroom door. You should also set aside some time to relax each day.

By closing your eyes, breathing deeply, and forgetting your `worries for a brief period, even if it's only 15 minutes a day, you can help reduce stress. Exercise will also help by giving you an outlet for the stress. Keeping your blood sugar level will also help.

2.   Tell Friends and Family that you're Dieting

By telling others that you're dieting, you have them to help keep you in check. Of course, you'll hear things like, "You're dieting aren't you" or "Are you supposed to be eating that," but it will help you stick to your diet. You'll also hear things like, "How much have you lost" or "You're looking so good." Those things can be very encouraging. Once you've made the proclamation that you're dieting, you'll feel like you have to prove you can do it, so you're more apt to stick with it and achieve success.

In addition, having a "buddy" system when you diet is a great way to lose weight. You have someone to help keep you in check, but you also have someone you can eat out with that you won't have to explain you're dieting to or someone that will be eating fattening foods in front of you. You can help and encourage each other along the way. You can celebrate each success you make as well as the success of your friends.

Trying to lose weight with a partner can help you stay accountable for your actions, as well as giving you an extra incentive to keep exercise appointments. Share your victories together, and discuss solutions to whatever roadblocks you encounter

3.   Don't Eat Sugar

Avoid Sugar-Sweetened Beverages Like the Plague. Added sugar is extremely unhealthy. Studies show that it has uniquely harmful effects on metabolic health. Sugar is half glucose, half fructose... and fructose can only be metabolized by the liver in any significant amount. When you eat a lot of refined sugar, the liver gets flooded with fructose, and is forced to turn it all into fat. Numerous studies have shown that excess sugar, mostly due to the large amounts of fructose, can lead to increased accumulation of fat in the belly. Some believe that this is the primary mechanism behind sugar's harmful effects on health... it increases belly fat and liver fat, which leads to insulin resistance and a host of metabolic problems. Liquid sugar is even worse in this regard. Liquid calories don't get "registered" by the brain in the same way as solid calories, so when you drink sugar-sweetened beverages, you end up eating more total calories. Studies show that sugar-sweetened beverages are linked to a 60% increased risk of obesity in children... per each daily serving. Make a decision to minimize the amount of sugar in your diet, and consider completely eliminating sugary drinks. This includes sugar-sweetened beverages, fruit juices, various sports drinks, as well as coffees and teas with sugar added to them. Keep in mind that none of this applies to whole fruit, which are extremely healthy and have plenty of fiber that mitigates the negative effects of fructose. The amount of fructose you get from fruit is negligible compared to what you get from a diet high in refined sugar. Btw... if you want to cut back on refined sugar, then you must start reading labels. Even foods marketed as health foods can contain huge amounts of sugar.

Summary: Excess sugar consumption may be the primary driver of belly fat accumulation, especially sugary beverages like soft drinks and fruit juices.

4.   Eating More Protein as the Best Long-Term Strategy for Reducing Belly Fat

Protein is the most important macronutrient when it comes to losing weight. It has been shown to reduce cravings by 60%, boost metabolism by 80-100 calories per day and help you eat up to 441 fewer calories per day. If weight loss is your goal, then adding protein to your diet is perhaps the single most effective change you can do. Not only will it help you lose... it can also help you avoid re-gaining weight if you ever decide to abandon your weight loss efforts. There is also some evidence that protein is particularly effective against belly fat. A study in Denmark showed that protein, especially animal protein, was linked to significantly reduced risk of belly fat gain over a period of 5 years. This study also showed that refined carbs and vegetable oils were linked to increased amounts of belly fat, but fruits and vegetables linked to reduced amounts. Many of the studies showing protein to be effective had protein at 25-30% of calories. That's what you should aim for.

Another study showed that the amount and quality of protein consumed was inversely related to fat in the belly. That is, people who ate more and better protein had much less belly fat.

So… make an effort to increase your intake of unprocessed eggs, fish, seafood, meats, poultry and dairy products. These are the best protein sources in the diet. If you struggle with getting enough protein in your diet, then a quality protein supplement (like whey protein) is a healthy and convenient way to boost your total intake.

Expert Advice: Consider cooking your foods in coconut oil… some studies have shown that 30 mL (about 2 tablespoons) of coconut oil per day reduces belly fat slightly.

Summary: Eating enough protein is a very effective way to lose weight. Some studies suggest that protein is particularly effective against belly fat accumulation.

5. Cut Carbs From Your Diet

Carb restriction is a very effective way to lose fat. This is supported by numerous studies… when people cut carbs, their appetite goes down and they lose weight. Over 20 randomized controlled trials have now shown that low-carb diets lead to 2-3 times more weight loss than low-fat diets.

This is true even when the low-carb groups are allowed to eat as much as they want, while the low-fat groups are calorie restricted and hungry. Low-carb diets also lead to quick reductions in water weight, which gives people near instant results… a major difference on the scale is often seen within a few days.

There are also studies comparing low-carb and low-fat diets, showing that low-carb diets specifically target the fat in the belly, and around the organs and liver. What this means is that a particularly high proportion of the fat lost on a low-carb diet is the dangerous and disease promoting abdominal fat. Just avoiding the refined carbs (white breads, pastas, etc.) should be sufficient, especially if you keep your protein high.

However… if you need to lose weight fast, then consider dropping your carbs down to 50 grams per day. This will put your body into ketosis, killing your appetite and making your body start burning primarily fats for fuel. Of course, low-carb diets have many other health benefits besides just weight loss. They can have life-saving effects in type 2 diabetics, for example.

Summary: Studies have shown that low-carb diets are particularly effective at getting rid of the fat in the belly area, around the organs and in the liver.

6.   Eat Foods Rich in Fiber… Especially Viscid Fiber

Dietary fiber is mostly indigestible plant matter. It is often claimed that eating plenty of fiber can help with weight loss. This is true… but it's important to keep in mind that not all fiber is created equal. It seems to be mostly the viscous fibers that can have an effect on your weight. These are fibers that bind water and form a thick gel that "sits" in the gut. This gel can dramatically slow the movement of food through your stomach and small bowel, and slow down the digestion and absorption of nutrients. The end result is a prolonged feeling of fullness and reduced appetite.

One review study found that an additional 14 grams of fiber per day were linked to a 10% decrease in calorie intake and weight loss of 2 kg (4.5 lbs) over 4 months. In one 5-year study, eating 10 grams of soluble fiber per day was linked to a 3.7% reduction in the amount of fat in the abdominal cavity, but it had no effect on the amount of fat under the skin.

What this implies, is that soluble fiber may be particularly effective at reducing the harmful belly fat.
The best way to get more fiber is to eat a lot of plant foods like vegetables and fruit. Legumes are also a good source, as well as some cereals like oats.

Summary: There is some evidence that soluble dietary fiber may lead to reduced amounts of belly fat, which should cause major improvements in metabolic health.

7.   Aerobic Exercise is Very Effective at Reducing Belly Fat

Exercise is important for various reasons. It is among the best things you can do if you want to live a long, healthy life and avoid disease. Getting into all of the amazing health benefits of exercise is not what this book is about, but exercise does appears to be effective at reducing belly fat.

Aerobics are a great way to get a good cardio workout. You can do this in a group, such as a class, or get an exercise video and do them in the privacy of your own home. Whichever way you choose, getting up your cardio rate will help your body burn fat. The exercise or dancing part of the aerobic exercise will help reduce fat and build muscle.

However... keep in mind that I'm not talking about abdominal exercises here. Spot reduction (losing fat in one spot) is not possible, and doing endless amounts of crunches will not make you lose fat from the belly.

In one study, 6 weeks of training just the abdominal muscles had no measurable effect on waist circumference or the amount of fat in the abdominal cavity. That being said, other types of exercise can be very effective. Aerobic exercise (like walking, running, swimming, etc.) has been shown to cause major reductions in belly fat in numerous studies.

Another study found that exercise completely prevented people from re-gaining abdominal fat after weight loss, implying that exercise is particularly important during weight maintenance. Exercise also leads to reduced inflammation, blood sugar levels and all the other metabolic abnormalities that are associated with central obesity.

Summary: Exercise can be very effective if you are trying to lose belly fat. Exercise also has a number of other health benefits.

8.   Track Your Foods and Figure Out What and How Much You Are Eating

What you eat is important. Pretty much everyone knows this. However... surprisingly, most people actually don't have a clue what they are really eating. People think they're eating "high protein," "low-carb" or whatever... but tend to drastically over- or underestimate. I think that for anyone who truly wants to optimize their diet, tracking things for a while is absolutely essential.

It doesn't mean you need to weigh and measure everything for the rest of your life, but doing it every now and then for a few days in a row can help you realize where you need to make changes.

If you want to boost your protein intake to 25-30% of calories, as recommended above, just eating more protein rich foods won't cut it. You need to actually measure and fine tune in order to reach that goal. I personally do this every few months… I weigh and measure everything I eat to see what my current diet is looking like. Then I know exactly where to make adjustments in order to get closer to my goals.

9.   Stop smoking and/or drinking

People often say if they stop smoking they'll gain weight and use that as an excuse to keep smoking. That is all it is…an excuse! Both smoking and drinking will cause you to gain weight and keep stubborn belly fat. Find something else to do with the time you usually spend smoking. Take short walks, exercise, or do something else that is healthy and good for your body instead of smoking which as you know is not a friend of your body.

10.   Eat

I know it may seem like an unreasonable measure, but it isn't. Eating is important when you're trying to reduce your weight, including trying to lose that resistant belly fat. Breakfast is very important when you're dieting. Many people will skip breakfast in an effort to lose weight, but that's one of the worst things you can do. Research has proven that eating about an hour after you get up from the bed can keep your insulin levels steadier and aid in keeping your weight steadier. You don't want to eat a whole chicken and two dozen eggs, but the consumption of breakfast that is high in fiber and protein can really boost your body metabolism and help you reduce fat.

It also makes more sense to eat 4 to 5 small meals a day than eat 1 or 2 large ones. Doing this you give signal to your body that it is going to get constant fuel. If you don't, or if you eat at irregular times and in irregular amounts, your body won't know it is going to be continually refueled. Your body reasons it has to store the fat for future energy use. Usually where does it store it…right around the midsection? You defeat the purpose of trying to lose belly fat if you don't eat in the morning.

11.   Don't Deep Fry

Often, people say they're "stir frying," but use so much oil that they might as well be deep frying their vegetables. Instead of using a lot of oil, just start with a drop of oil. Then, gradually add water and let the vegetables stir-fry in their own moisture. Studies have shown that this does not only reduces your fat intake, it actually gives the vegetables a better taste.

12.   Heat your skillet when you fry

If you heat your skillet first before adding the oil, the oil gets hot quicker and less oil will be assimilated by your food. But if you put oil in a cold skillet, and add vegetables or meats, the food will get soaked. If it soaks into the food, where does it go? It goes right into your body and adds to belly fat.

13. Fake your Food

Sometimes, it isn't how much you eat that makes you full, it's how much you "think" you've eaten. When you have a flat small piece of meat on your plate that is truly small, it seems like you've been deprived. If you cut this same meat thinly and stack it on your plate, surprisingly, it appears to be a bigger portion, so you think you've eaten more. This works for fruits and vegetables as well. A small ham sliced up will look larger. You'll think you're eating more than you really are.

14. Marinade without oil

Marinating in oil leads to the food being soaked with oil, so naturally, it will be eaten. One recipe for oil-free marinade is to combine apple juice (about 3 cups) pressed garlic (2 cloves) and soy sauce that is reduced sodium (about 1 cup). Marinating in a healthy manner can greatly reduce the amount of fat you intake.

15. Stuff your Food

If you fill the heart or core of your food with wholesome ingredients, you'll be eating as much food, but reducing your caloric intake. One great example is to stuff your food with oats. Use oats that are of the same proportion with the same amount of other things you use in filling, such as crackers or bread crumbs. Not only are oats better for you, because they have high fiber content, they taste the same, and can help you reduce your cholesterol. Check out the following examples:

• Take your hamburger and put a hole in the center of the meat before you cook it. Fill it with some type of vegetables such as: mushrooms, olives, or anything else you like. If you use the recommended serving size of three ounces, you will succeed in making it look much bigger, more filling, and much leaner. Imagine if what you added instead of the vegetables is the same amount of hamburger to make it that size, then you would have been successful in making it much less healthy.

• Do you want to add vitamins and moisture as well as size to your meatballs without changing the flavor? Then fill up your meatballs with grated carrots or squash. By doing this you will be able to make your meatballs bigger, and not add calories and fat.

16. Make a Food Swap

Most times you can speed up your belly fat reduction process by substituting something healthier for something full of fat in your favorite recipes. By doing that, you'll be preventing that fat from settling in your belly and reducing that dreaded fat. Start with the following changes:

• When you prepare your curry, use plain yogurt rather than coconut milk which is full of fat. You'll get a good, creamy texture, but you won't have all the fat.

• Trade two slices of bread for one piece of pita bread— folding a piece of pita bread will allow you to put more vegetables on your sandwich. More vegetables make it more filling, and you'll succeed in making a healthier sandwich.

• Supplant red meat with lentils—in foods such as lasagna, only use about half the amount of ground beef. Use red lentil in filling because it is packed with protein. It is fat-free, and high in fiber. Its flavor is neutral, so it will just absorb the flavor of your sauce and you won't notice the difference.

• Consume the "turkey" versions of your favorite meat—you can have turkey ham, turkey burger, turkey hot dogs, or even turkey pepperoni. Turkey isn't near as high in fat as other meats. You'll have the flavor of the other meats without that added fat to carry around.

17. Change your Toppings

If you must have toppings on your food, consider adding at least two vegetable toppings. If you do this for every meat ordered as a topping, you'll have a healthier food. The cancer causing agents in processed meats have been found to increase the risk of cancer, so you'll not only be reducing your belly fat, you'll be improving your health.

Also reduce cheese in your toppings. If you have a recipe that requires a grated cheese topping, you can bust fat and add fiber by replacing half of the cheese with whole-wheat bread crumbs. The crumbs keep the texture of the baked cheese, so you won't know the difference.

18.   Replace "fish-n-chips" with healthier, low-fat recipe

Use white fish such as cod or haddock and cut it in pieces. Use sparkling water and self-rising flour for a light batter mix. Fry the cut pieces in a small amount of canola oil. Instead of deep fried French fries, rather use cut potatoes baked at 450 degrees in canola oil and seasoned with herbs, salt, garlic, etc.

19.   Eat Healthier Deli Meat

Not all Deli meats are bad; you just need to learn to eat the healthier ones. In order of health, first would be chicken or turkey. Second is roast beef. Third is ham. Lastly, we have all the other processed deli meats such as bologna, salami, olive loaf, etc.

20.   Don't Suffocate your Food

It's no fun to eat what you can't even see, so don't drown your food! Don't drown your food in catsup or mayo or goo. How many times has it happened that someone prepares a nice, healthy salad only to add so much fattening dressing that it's no longer healthy? Some people will also add so much sauce that a lean piece of roast turkey becomes unhealthy. Make your toppings instead of extra virgin olive oil that is seasoned on salads. This will keep your food healthy and won't sacrifice the taste.

21.   Do away with Fattening Mayonnaise

If you must add anything to your tuna fish choose to add hot sauce, lemon juice, and pepper. It tastes great and adds no fat.

22.   Cheat once a Week

Use the meal as a reward for a week's worth of hard work, or the completion of a project you've been dreading. "It's OK for people to blow one meal a week without feeling guilty," a food researcher said. "If you follow a healthy diet 95% of the time, you can relax and enjoy yourself the other 5% of the time without gaining weight," he added.

23.   Use grated cheese instead of slices

When you use grate hard cheeses such as Parmesan on your sandwiches you'll get the entire cheese flavor with much less fat.

24.   Eat your meals without meat

I'm not saying go totally Vegan, but every meal doesn't have to be a "meat and potato" meal. Eat vegetarian lasagna without adding beef. Consume eggplant parmesan instead of veal parmesan. You'll be taking in less fat, so there'll be less fat to stay around your midsection.

25.   Replace Cheese with squash

Squash is embedded with a high proportion of vitamins and potassium, so not only will your food have less fat and calories, it will be healthier. By adding pureed butternut squash to half the cheese mixture in foods like macaroni and cheese, quesadillas, or grilled sandwiches will greatly bust the calorie count without altering the taste of the food.

26.   Wrap your Meat in Greens

Wrap your meat in a large lettuce leaf or some other leafy green such as romaine lettuce, or Chinese cabbage rather than eating meats that are between two slices of bread. You'll be reducing your intake of carbs that can add belly fat.

27.   Use Avocados rather than Mayonnaise

Research suggest that a diet with a higher ratio of monounsaturated fats like avocados, nuts, seeds, soybeans, and chocolate — can prevent the accumulation of belly fat. Ripe avocados will make your sandwich moist like mayonnaise, and have good fat instead of bad fat. This can also lower your cholesterol. Trans-fats (in margarines, crackers, cookies, or anything made with partially hydrogenated oils) seem to result in more fat being deposited in the abdomen. Avoid these as much as possible.

28.   Make your pancakes healthier

Cornmeal is healthier than traditional flour. It has a higher fiber content, as well as magnesium. For healthier pancakes, replace half your flour with cornmeal. They'll have a great texture and be better for you.

29. Pucker up

Obese people who consumed a tablespoon or two of vinegar daily for eight weeks showed significant decreases in body fat, particularly visceral fat, according to a 2009 Japanese study. "One theory is that the acetic acid in the vinegar produces proteins that burn up fat," explains Pamela Peeke, professor of medicine at the University of Maryland and author of "Fight Fat After 40".

Studies show that acidic foods such as vinegar and lemon juice work like lighter fluid in your body's fat incinerator, increasing carb combustion 20%-40%. Researchers believe the acids blunt insulin spikes and slow the rate at which food empties from your stomach. Fermented foods like pickles and yogurt are also good sour options. So, learn to top your salad with vinaigrette dressing.

30. Endeavor to get all the Vitamins Available in your Cereal

If you've taken the steps to eat healthier breakfast cereals, you probably aren't getting all the nutrition from it that you should. In order to do so, you need to drink the milk in the bowl. As much as 40 percent of the nutritional vitamins from your cereal will dissolve into the milk, so drinking it makes it healthier for you.

31. Take Frozen Bananas

Frozen bananas are great for making smoothies that are healthy and nutritious. They're sweet, so they eliminate the need for sugary ingredients. Frozen, they have the cold state for good thick smoothies and won't go bad quickly like they can if they're unfrozen.

32. Eat chocolate

Yes, you read correctly. So often, people ignore their cravings for chocolate because they feel it is "bad" for them. Dark chocolate, however, is lower in fat and very high in antioxidants, so eating it will both satisfy your cravings and give you a healthy snack. You can also shave dark chocolate into dishes like barbecue sauce or chili. It gives it a good flavor boost, and will help you prevent heart disease as well as keep your cholesterol at a good level. If you want a good night-time snack, take two tablespoons of dark chocolate and melt it in the microwave. Stir it with 4 ounces of vanilla yogurt and top it with about a tablespoon of almond slivers.

33.   Make your dips yourself

Dips bought in shops can be very high in fat and calories. But if you make your dips yourself, however, you can greatly reduce the fat and calories. Just use fat-free sour cream or yogurt. You can mix it with an equal portion of salsa or add herbs and/or lemon. Whatever flavor you choose will be much healthier for you this way.

34.   Go for Shelled Nuts

.Nuts in and of themselves can be healthy, especially pistachios, almonds and walnuts. If, however, you eat too many, they become like any other food and will cause you to gain weight. If you have to spend time shelling the nuts, you'll spend less time eating big handfuls of them.

35.   Boil your Peanuts

Boiled peanuts are a popular snack already in Asia, China, Australia, and the southern portion of the US. If you haven't tried them, the next time you want peanuts, give them a try. Studies have shown that if peanuts are boiled for a few hours, they will have approximately four times the amount of antioxidants when they are prepared any other way.

Nuts have a very high satiety power—meaning they make you feel fuller after eating than many other foods. And even though they're high in calories, those calories appear to be processed differently in the body. University of Michigan researchers found that men who added 500 calories' worth of peanuts a day to their diet gained no excess weight at all.

36.   Snack First

If you're going out for a business dinner or to a party of some kind, eat a healthy, high-protein snack before you go. This will make you less hungry, and will allow you to eat smaller portions of the more fattening foods. This not only keeps you from being ravenous—and overeating—at lunch and dinner, it forces your body to process food all day long, which keeps your metabolism stoked.

37.   Even your baked potatoes

Many people do away with baked potatoes because of the high glycemic rating. You can have them, however, you must balance them with a healthy topping like cheddar cheese, broccoli, mushrooms, or spinach.

38. Rinse your Canned Beans

Beans such as kidney beans are a great way to add both fiber and protein to a meal. Canned beans, however, contain a lot of sodium. This can give you a bloated feeling as well as cause high blood pressure. Rinsing them, however, washes away that high sodium content and makes them healthy again.

39. Thicken your Side Dishes

There is a way by which you can give your food a thicker texture. Using evaporated milk that is fat-free in dishes like mashed potatoes or macaroni and cheese, give them a thicker texture that will seem more filling. In addition to that, you'll be taking in more calcium per cup without all the fat.

40. Drink Plenty of Water

Water is filling, cleansing, and keeps you properly hydrated. If you drink two glasses of water before each meal, you will fill up quicker and eat less. The water will take up room in your stomach, making you feel fuller and reducing your appetite, says Christopher Mohr, M.S., R.D.

Moreover, studies suggest that consistently drinking water throughout the day can lead to a more active metabolism, regardless of dieting. Drinking more water also helps your body flush out waste/toxins and improves your overall health. Aim to drink an 8-oz. glass of water 8 times per day, or 64 ounces total. Carry a water bottle so that you can drink whenever you feel thirsty.

How do you tell when you're adequately hydrated? You'll know you're drinking enough water when your urine runs almost clear. If it's still colored yellow, drink up. Significantly reduce alcohol, sugary drinks (like Coke, 7-Up, Pepsi and all the diet drinks), and carbonated beverages.

Alcohol is another cause of bloat since it causes dehydration, which can lead to water retention. For your health and your belly's sake, stick to one alcoholic beverage if you must, and follow it with a huge glass of water.

41. Spice up your Life

Research has proven that overweight people will become slimmer if they eat meals that contain Chili peppers. They contain capsaicin. It's what makes them hot, and it helps the liver clear insulin from your bloodstream after you eat. Since insulin is the hormone that tells your body to store the fat, clearing it from the body can reduce belly fat.

42. Don't do Emotional Eating

When you feel like eating just to eat and you know you're not hungry, substitute it with something else like going on a bike. If you must eat something, make it fresh fruits or vegetables. Do not engage in the practice of using food to comfort yourself. When you're hurt or upset, you turn to food to make you feel better. Don't do it.

BELLY EXERCISES

While exercise is an essential part of weight loss, you should realize that exercises that target your abdominal area won't help you burn the fat. They will define the muscles there, but in order to achieve that abs, you first have to get rid of all the fat you have in your belly. Here are a few tips you can use to exercise your way to less belly fat:

43. Walk

Endeavor to get in at least 10,000 steps each and every day. If you have a sedentary job, this may be difficult for you. Schedule a time and place to do brisk walking every day. If you can't, then choose a few other walking activities like parking at the far end of the parking lot at work or when you go to grocery or department stores. Take the steps instead of the elevator.

44. Ramp up the Cardio

Engage in aerobic exercises which get your heart pumping. It also burn calories quickly and leads to fat loss all over the body, not excluding your belly. You can't "spot-burn" belly fat, but it's usually the first to burn off when you exercise, regardless of body shape or size.

Track your progress: Track your progress by timing how long it takes to run a mile. As cardiovascular stamina improves, you'll notice the time going down.

Correct shin splints: If you get painful shin splints (pain along the front of your shins when you run), you may be over-pronating (landing with most of your weight on the outer side of your foot). There are shoes designed specifically to help eliminate or reduce this.

Don't overdo it: When first getting into cardio, aim to workout 2 or maybe 3 days a week, then build up to 4 when you're able. Pushing yourself too hard doesn't allow your body enough time to recover and build up muscle, and could lead to injury.

45.　Go on a bike

Bike riding at a cardio pace, is a great way to get a good workout and burn calories. Many people who are too busy to do a workout should get their exercise from biking to and from work each day. You can jump start your metabolism each morning with a good ride, and then reduce stress of a hectic day on the ride home. Biking is both a stress remedy and a fat burner.

46.　Jog

Not everybody can get involved in jogging. Many people stay fit and trim by jogging. This can be done outdoors, on an indoor track, or on a treadmill. If your age is 50 and above, you want to check with your physician to be sure you're physically fit for jogging. Many times the jar from jogging on the knees, hips, and/or back can be harmful to those with problems. Once you've got a clean bill of health, "run, run and keep running!"

47.　Take a Martial Arts Class

Martial arts classes are good for cardio workouts, muscle definition, and self-defense. Asians have long used this to trim and reduce body fat. Martial arts can also be a lot of fun. If you're finding it difficult to join a class alone, talk a friend into joining with you.

48.　Weight Training or Pilates

When either of Pilates or weight training is done together with a good cardio workout, can help you build muscle. Muscle will burn calories. You can find free weight training workouts for beginners to advanced, and Pilates classes are available for all levels as well. Cardio work out 2 to 5 times a week with a good weight training program will help you burn overall body fat including that dreaded belly fat.

49. Breath Control Exercises

One good form of auxiliary exercise is breath control exercises that are good for the abdominal region. Yoga is a leading example. Though it is not compulsory, and not vital for reducing belly fat, it is a simple way to strengthen the abdominal area and remove inches from your waistline.

Postmenopausal women who tried yoga for 16 weeks reported significant reductions in visceral fat in one 2012 study. If you're just not that into downward dog, any sort of relaxation exercise, even simple deep breathing, can help—the key is to lower the levels of the stress hormone cortisol, which is linked to belly fat.

50. Maintain Good Posture

Although you might not be aware, but the truth remains that you use many core muscles simply to hold yourself up straight in good posture. The maintenance of good posture while tightening the stomach muscles can strengthen both the back muscles and the abdominal muscles.

51. Exercise in Small Bursts

Research has revealed that alternating bursts of energy, that is one, small ones, with brief resting periods can not only improve your muscle tone and burn calories, but it can also build endurance. This is a good way to get started and build up to the more serious exercises. You might attempt running. Just run as fast as you can for around 20 seconds. Walk until your breathing returns to normal, and do it again. If you do this for about 10 minutes a day, you'll be on your way to a good start.

Set your exercise equipment for interval training—in this mode, it increases the difficulty for short periods and then returns to normal. It gives you the effect of exercising in small bursts by using machines.

52. Fit some type of exercise into your normal work day

Work can sometimes be very tedious and difficult for some people. It depends on the type of job you have. You might sacrifice your lunch hours for walking. If that's not possible, plan 7 minutes out of each day for a power walk. Take long, brisk strides when you walk down the hall or go up and down stairs.

53. Stretch the Sides of your waist

With one arm over your head lean as far as you can to the opposite side. Then switch hands. This will strengthen the muscles of your waistline. It will tone them, and remember, muscle burns fat, so having good muscle tone is important.

54. Simple leg lifts

To tighten the abdominal muscles, lay flat on your back. Raise your feet about two inches off the ground and hold it while you slow count to ten. Lower your feet and then do it again. Try to do this at least 10 times a daily. It is a simple basic way to begin to strengthen weakened abdominal muscles.

55. When all else Fails, there's always Surgery

If you've tried everything and you just can't get rid of your belly fat, there are two types of surgery you could consider.

- **Tummy tuck**—this is also referred to as an abdominoplasty. It takes out the excess fat and skin you have stored in your midsection. It can usually reestablish weakened muscles which gives you an abdominal area that is firmer.

- **Panniculectomy**—this can be done by itself or along with an abdominoplasty. It removes any overhanging skin and tissue known as an "apron" from below the naval. This skin usually occurs when people have had excessive weight loss.

If you have overhanging skin, it can cause you a lot of problems. Obviously, it would pull on your back, causing back pain. It can also cause hygiene problems, and yeast infections. Sometimes cysts develop in the folds. If you have this overhanging skin, it shouldn't be ignored.

Though people may be happy with their inner selves and with who they are as a person, not many people will say they're happy about being overweight. If you're unhappy with yourselves, it's time to get motivated to lose the weight. If you want to lose weight and keep it off, you'll need a lot of motivation. It isn't just about going on a diet. It's a complete, total lifestyle change. You've had the habits of overeating for a long time. It takes time to get rid of those habits and establish new ones. Once you've established the new ones, however, you can begin shedding that belly fat.

Remember, losing the weight is only half the battle. Keeping the weight off can often be harder than losing it. If you want to keep it off, you have to make a commitment to a lifestyle change. If you go back to your old habits, you can gain all the weight you lost and more. You have to find new eating habits that you can live with.
They have to be habits you can sustain for a lifetime.

Make sure you keep your regimen of healthy eating and exercise. Even if you opt for tip 55 and have surgery, the weight can still return.

If motivation is difficult for you, find someone who can give you support and encourage you. It may be your doctor, your spouse, a friend or another family member. This often helps you stay on track.

Sometimes it's hard to make lifestyle changes that suit us. They need to go along with our physical fitness and overall state of health. You want to be sure to talk to your doctor. He/she can help you weigh all the options and decide what plan of action works best for you. Your goal is to have long-term success. You may have to try different options to find out what works for you.

Sometimes, in your weight-loss process, you may get stuck. You lose a certain amount of weight and just can't lose any more. It's important not to give up. You've set a weight-loss goal, and you want to reach it. In order to do so, sometimes all you have to do is make a few minor changes to what you're doing. You can reduce your calories a bit or increase your exercise. Walk an extra mile. Whatever you can find that gives you that push over the edge and jump starts you again. Whatever you do, don't give up. You'll get excited about seeing your waistline reduce and be motivated to press on. If you get stuck, however, it can be a bit disheartening.

Sometimes, you may be motivated by health improvements. You can check your cholesterol levels. If they decrease, you know you're reducing your changes of heart disease. You may see a regular blood pressure for the first time in years. Your breathing may improve and you'll be able to do a lot more than you used to. These things are motivators to keep the weight off for many people. If you're losing weight for health reasons, however, note that sometimes it takes a while for these interventions to kick in.

You didn't become unhealthy overnight, and losing a few pounds isn't going to instantly change that. It is a gradual process, so keep pressing forward. Eventually, you'll see the results.

It is important to remember that you may not be able to lose weight the way your Great Aunt Ruth did. You may go on a diet with a friend and they may lose and you may not. Remember that you didn't gain the weight at the same rate or by eating and doing exactly the same thing. All bodies are different. They work in different ways. What works for you might not work for your friends either. You have to find something that works for YOU! Don't stop until you've found something. Get to know your own body and how it works. That will help you find the right solution and combination of foods and exercises that works best for you.

Know that doing 100 crunches a day for the rest of your life won't reduce your belly fat. Too many people believe that and are greatly disappointed when they work that hard and have nothing to show for it. You have to reduce your intake of processed carbohydrates and eat fat-burning proteins instead.

For unknown reasons, belly fat just seems to burn slower than the fat on the rest of your body. You didn't get that belly overnight, and you won't lose it overnight either. The good news is, however, that it does burn! It may take a few weeks to see progress, but keep it up and you will see it.

It isn't easy to lose weight and then keep it off. If you've accomplished this, it is an important achievement. You probably feel good about yourself, but don't be surprised if you find that you are better able to face other challenges and also succeed in them. Sometimes eating healthier is easier than exercising. One good tip to keep exercising is if you're having a bad day and you don't feel like exercising, go halfway. Get in your car and go to the gym. Once you get there, you might not want to go in. That's fine. At least driving yourself there is a step. Usually, you'll think, "Well, I'm here, I might as well go in." Once you do, those endorphins kick in and you find yourself enjoying the exercise and greatly benefiting from it.

As you go along, you can actually measure your progress using what is known as your "waist-to-hip" ratio. To do this, you measure the narrowest part of your waist and the broadest portion of your hips. Then you divide the circumference of your waistline by the circumference of your hips. Just divide the waist measurement by the hip measurement. A woman should have a ratio that is 0.8 or lower. A man should have a ratio of 0.9 or lower.

Don't rely on your memory. Actually write down your progress. Keep all your measurements written down together some place so you can easily chart your progress as you go. This can be a big encouragement and motivator to keep going. When you're measuring, make sure you weigh yourself at the same time of the day each time. Weight can fluctuate during different parts of the day. This can be predicted by your last meal or your last bowel movement. By measuring at the same time of the day, you'll get a better idea of your true weight loss. Most people find in the morning before breakfast as the best time.

When you feel yourself having difficulty being motivated to exercise, try putting forth half of the effort. At least get in your car and go over to the gym. You can always turn around and go home if you don't feel like it once you get there. Chances are, however, you'll feel, "I've made it this far, I might as well go in and give exercising a try." Don't commit to a full exercise routine. Just commit to working on the bicycle for 10 minutes. Once you do that, you can commit to one more thing at a time until you finish. If, however, you don't feel like it, at least you can say you tried. Once those endorphins kick in, however, you'll probably feel like it.
You'll probably feel much better when you're finished.

If you're really tired of belly fat and desperate to lose weight, don't take those desperate measures some people take. They starve themselves, try every fad diet that comes out, or take expensive supplements that don't work just because they all say you will lose weight immediately. Losing that belly fat just isn't going to happen overnight. Yo-yo dieting will only mess up your body's metabolism and cause you to gain more weight than you lost in the first place. Starving causes you to binge at the first temptation of something you love to eat. Your system gets so confused, it's no wonder that belly fat stays.

Keeping your body's metabolism running effectively and continuously burning calories is what will help you prevent that fat storage around your midsection and keep you from gaining weight again. When you eat healthy foods and exercise you'll develop lean muscle mass which will allow you to intake calories and not gain weight because muscle helps burn fat.

Don't forget as you begin the weight-loss process, you need to set realistic goals. If your goals aren't realistic and achievable, then you'll become discouraged. You'll lose confidence in yourself and give up easier. Setting realistic goals will help give you that boost of confidence you each time you reach one to move forward in your weight loss.